AF688021

AI Injury Prediction & Sports Medicine

How Smart Systems Detect Risk Before Athletes Break

By Joe Correa

Published by Live Stronger Faster

Copyright © 2026 by Joe Correa

All rights reserved.

No part of this publication may be reproduced, distributed, or transmitted in any form or by any means—electronic, mechanical, photocopying, recording, or otherwise—without the prior written permission of the publisher, except in the case of brief quotations embodied in critical reviews and certain other noncommercial uses permitted by copyright law.

This book is for educational and informational purposes only. The author and publisher are not engaged in rendering legal, financial, or other professional advice. Readers should consult a qualified professional before making any financial decisions.

First Edition

Table of Contents

Introduction

Modern sports medicine is undergoing one of the most profound transformations in history as artificial intelligence moves injury prevention from reactive treatment to proactive prediction. For decades, athletes and medical professionals relied on pain signals, visible breakdowns, or catastrophic events to indicate injury risk. By the time an athlete felt discomfort, damage had often already begun. AI changes this paradigm entirely by identifying subtle physiological, biomechanical, and neurological signals that indicate risk days, weeks, or even months before an injury occurs. This shift allows athletes to modify training loads, movement patterns, and recovery protocols before breakdown happens, preserving performance and extending careers.

At the core of AI-driven injury prediction is data aggregation. Modern athletes generate enormous volumes of data from training sessions, games, wearables, motion-capture systems, force plates, heart-rate monitors, sleep trackers, and even psychological stress assessments. AI systems are uniquely capable of integrating these disparate data streams into a single predictive model. Instead of evaluating one metric in isolation, such as mileage or weight lifted, AI evaluates patterns across thousands of variables simultaneously. Small deviations—slight asymmetries in stride, changes in muscle activation timing, or declining recovery efficiency—are identified as early warning signs that human observers would almost certainly miss.

Machine learning models improve injury prediction accuracy by learning from historical injury data. By analyzing thousands or even millions of athlete profiles, AI systems learn which patterns most commonly precede specific injuries such as ACL tears, hamstring strains, rotator cuff damage, or stress fractures. These models are continuously refined as new data is collected, meaning prediction accuracy improves over time. Unlike static risk assessments, AI systems adapt to the individual athlete, adjusting predictions based on age, position, injury history, workload tolerance, and even genetics when available.

Biomechanical analysis plays a critical role in AI-based injury prevention. High-speed cameras and motion sensors capture joint angles, force distribution, and movement timing with extreme precision. AI evaluates how efficiently force travels through the kinetic chain during movement. Even minor inefficiencies—such as delayed hip activation or excessive knee valgus—can compound under repetitive stress. AI identifies these inefficiencies early and recommends corrective strategies, allowing athletes to adjust mechanics before tissue overload leads to injury. Load management is another area where AI dramatically reduces injury risk. Overtraining remains one of the leading causes of athletic breakdown, often due to a mismatch between workload and recovery capacity. AI systems analyze acute-to-chronic workload ratios, recovery markers, sleep quality, hormonal signals, and nervous system readiness to determine how much stress an athlete can safely tolerate. Instead of following rigid training schedules, AI enables dynamic programming that adjusts volume and intensity in real time, ensuring athletes remain within optimal adaptation zones.

AI-driven sports medicine also enhances rehabilitation protocols. When injuries do occur, AI systems track healing progress with unprecedented precision. Sensor data and movement analysis allow AI to assess tissue readiness, neuromuscular coordination, and psychological confidence during rehab exercises. This prevents both premature return to play, which increases reinjury risk, and unnecessary delays that can erode performance. Rehab becomes a data-guided progression rather than a time-based estimate, leading to safer and faster recoveries.

Psychological stress is increasingly recognized as a major contributor to injury risk, and AI systems are now capable of integrating mental and emotional data into injury prediction models. Elevated stress levels alter movement patterns, increase muscle tension, and impair recovery. AI analyzes mood surveys, sleep disruptions, heart rate variability, and behavioral data to detect when mental strain may increase physical vulnerability. By addressing psychological factors alongside physical ones, AI provides a more holistic injury prevention strategy.

At the elite level, professional teams use AI injury prediction systems to guide roster decisions, practice planning, and in-game substitutions. Coaches receive real-time risk assessments that inform whether an athlete should be rested, limited, or removed from competition. This data-driven approach reduces emotionally driven decisions and protects athletes from short-term risk in pursuit of long-term performance sustainability. Increasingly, similar tools are becoming available to collegiate, amateur, and even youth athletes, democratizing access to elite-level sports medicine insights.

Ethical considerations play an important role in AI sports medicine adoption. Data privacy, informed consent, and transparent communication are essential to ensure athletes trust the systems designed to protect them. When used responsibly, AI empowers athletes rather than controls them. The most effective implementations emphasize collaboration between AI systems, medical professionals, coaches, and athletes, ensuring decisions are guided by data but grounded in human judgment.

Ultimately, AI injury prediction represents a fundamental shift in how sports view health and performance. Instead of reacting to breakdowns, athletes now operate within intelligent systems designed to preserve resilience, optimize readiness, and extend peak performance windows. As AI technology continues to evolve, injury prevention will become increasingly precise, personalized, and proactive—turning fragility into durability and uncertainty into confidence.

Ethan didn't just stay healthy, he got faster

Ethan had always believed injuries were part of the game. As a professional sprinter chasing fractions of a second, he accepted pain as the cost of speed. Tight hamstrings, sore hips, and aching calves were just background noise in his pursuit of personal records. But after his second hamstring tear in two seasons, his confidence began to crack. The injury didn't just take his speed—it stole his trust in his own body.

When his training facility introduced an AI-driven injury prediction system, Ethan was skeptical. He had worked with world-class trainers and doctors before. What could an algorithm possibly see that they hadn't? Still, with his career hanging in the balance, he agreed to participate. Sensors were attached during training sessions, cameras tracked his sprints, and wearables monitored everything from sleep quality to nervous system recovery.

Within weeks, the AI system flagged something unexpected. Ethan wasn't injured—but he was trending toward one. The system identified subtle asymmetries in his stride during maximum acceleration and a delayed firing pattern in his left glute. Combined with increasing nervous system fatigue and reduced sleep efficiency, the AI calculated a high probability of hamstring strain within the next three weeks if training continued unchanged.

At first, Ethan resisted the recommendations. The AI suggested reducing sprint volume temporarily and adding targeted neuromuscular drills. To him, backing off felt like weakness. But his coach showed him the data—clear visualizations of force imbalances and recovery decline. Reluctantly, Ethan agreed to follow the plan.

The changes were small but precise. His workouts were adjusted daily based on readiness scores. Recovery sessions were optimized for nervous system reset rather than just muscle soreness. Movement drills retrained firing sequences he didn't even realize were off. Over time, Ethan felt something he hadn't felt in years—confidence without fear. As the season progressed, Ethan didn't just stay healthy. He got faster. The AI system continued to monitor his risk levels, constantly adapting his program. For the first time, he wasn't guessing how hard to push or when to rest. The uncertainty that once haunted him was replaced by clarity.

At the national championships, Ethan lined up at the blocks feeling calm. Not reckless. Not desperate. Just ready. He exploded out of the start, his stride smooth and powerful. When he crossed the finish line, the scoreboard flashed a personal best. No pain. No hesitation. Just performance.

Later that night, Ethan reviewed his season data with his coach. The AI system had predicted three potential injury windows throughout the year—all of which were avoided through early intervention. For Ethan, the realization was profound. The technology hadn't replaced his intuition; it had protected it. It allowed him to train with confidence instead of fear.

As he prepared for the next phase of his career, Ethan understood something fundamental had changed. Injuries were no longer an inevitable cost of ambition. With AI as a silent partner, his body wasn't something to gamble with—it was something to understand. And that understanding gave him the greatest competitive edge he had ever known.

Chapter 1

From Reactive Treatment to Predictive Protection

For most of sports history, injuries have been treated as unavoidable interruptions rather than predictable outcomes. Athletes trained, competed, broke down, and then sought medical care only after pain or dysfunction appeared. This reactive model shaped generations of sports medicine, where diagnosis followed damage and recovery began only after loss had already occurred. Artificial intelligence is now dismantling this outdated framework by transforming injury prevention into a predictive science, allowing athletes and medical professionals to identify risk before tissues fail.

The fundamental shift introduced by AI is the ability to detect invisible precursors to injury. Human clinicians rely heavily on symptoms, visual assessments, and athlete feedback, all of which occur late in the injury timeline. AI systems, by contrast, identify microscopic deviations in movement, neuromuscular timing, force distribution, and recovery patterns long before discomfort emerges. These deviations are not random; they are early indicators of biomechanical overload, neuromuscular fatigue, and systemic stress accumulation. AI recognizes these patterns not through intuition, but through continuous analysis of high-resolution data streams.

Injury risk is rarely the result of a single variable. Instead, it emerges from the interaction of workload, recovery capacity, biomechanics, psychological stress, and environmental factors. AI excels in this complexity. By integrating training volume, intensity, sleep quality, heart rate variability, hormonal indicators, movement symmetry, and historical injury data, AI constructs a dynamic risk profile unique to each athlete. This individualized model evolves daily, reflecting the athlete's current readiness rather than relying on static benchmarks or generic injury thresholds.

Machine learning allows AI systems to improve injury prediction accuracy over time. Each training session, competition, and recovery period adds new data that refines predictive models. These systems learn which combinations of variables most frequently precede specific injuries. For example, a slight decrease in hamstring eccentric strength combined with increased sprint volume and reduced sleep efficiency may signal elevated strain risk. AI does not merely flag these patterns—it quantifies their probability, allowing medical teams to intervene with precision rather than speculation. One of the most powerful contributions of AI injury prediction is its ability to separate productive stress from harmful overload. Athletic adaptation requires pushing the body beyond comfort zones, but the margin between optimal stress and injury risk is narrow. Traditional training programs often rely on standardized progression models that fail to account for individual variability. AI continuously recalibrates this margin by monitoring how each athlete responds to stress. When adaptation slows or recovery markers decline, AI recommends adjustments that preserve progress while reducing risk.

Biomechanics serve as a central pillar of predictive injury analysis. Advanced motion capture systems feed AI precise data on joint angles, acceleration patterns, force absorption, and coordination timing. Even subtle compensations—often undetectable to coaches—can significantly increase injury risk when repeated thousands of times. AI identifies these inefficiencies early and connects them to underlying causes such as fatigue, mobility restrictions, or neuromuscular inhibition. This allows corrective strategies to be implemented before structural damage occurs.

Psychological and neurological factors also play a critical role in injury vulnerability. Stress, anxiety, and cognitive fatigue alter motor control, increase muscle tension, and impair recovery. AI systems incorporate psychological assessments, sleep disruptions, and nervous system indicators into injury prediction models. This holistic approach acknowledges that the brain is not separate from the body but an active participant in injury risk. By addressing mental load alongside physical stress, AI enables more complete protection strategies.

The transition from reactive treatment to predictive protection represents a philosophical shift in sports culture. Athletes no longer wait for warning signs; they operate within intelligent systems designed to anticipate breakdown. This does not eliminate risk entirely, but it dramatically reduces preventable injuries while extending athletic longevity. AI becomes not a replacement for medical expertise, but an amplifier—enhancing human judgment with continuous, objective insight.

As AI injury prediction becomes more accessible, its impact extends beyond elite sports. Youth athletes, recreational competitors, and aging populations benefit from systems that prioritize durability over short-term output. The future of sports medicine is not about fixing broken athletes—it is about preventing them from breaking in the first place. This chapter establishes the foundation for understanding how AI makes that future possible.

The Warning Before the Pain

Marcus had never considered himself injury-prone. As a professional soccer midfielder, he prided himself on durability. While teammates rotated through the training room, Marcus logged minutes, seasons, and miles without complaint. So when his club introduced an AI-based injury prediction platform, he viewed it as something meant for fragile players—not someone like him.

The system was introduced quietly at first. Training vests with embedded sensors. Cameras mounted above the pitch. Sleep and recovery questionnaires that fed into a centralized dashboard. Marcus participated without much thought, answering questions and wearing equipment as instructed. He trained hard, pushed harder, and felt fine—at least on the surface.

Three weeks into the season, the alert came. The AI flagged Marcus as "high risk" for a lower-leg overuse injury within fourteen days if his training load remained unchanged. Marcus laughed when the performance coach showed him the report. No pain. No stiffness. No warning signs. He had played through worse conditions than this.

But the data told a different story. The system had detected subtle asymmetries in Marcus's deceleration patterns and a gradual decline in neuromuscular recovery. His heart rate variability showed elevated stress, and his sleep data revealed fragmented rest after intense match days. Individually, none of these metrics were alarming. Together, they formed a pattern the AI recognized immediately.

The medical staff proposed a minor adjustment—slightly reduced high-intensity volume, targeted recovery sessions, and movement re-patterning drills. Marcus resisted. He didn't want to lose his starting spot or appear weak. But after reviewing injury timelines from similar athletes, he reluctantly agreed.

Over the next two weeks, Marcus felt something unexpected. He didn't feel slower. He felt sharper. His legs responded better late in matches. His recovery improved. The tightness he had subconsciously ignored faded without ever becoming pain. When the AI system downgraded his risk status, Marcus began to understand what had almost happened.

Later that season, a teammate who dismissed a similar warning suffered a stress fracture that sidelined him for months. Watching from the stands, Marcus felt a chill. He realized the injury hadn't come suddenly—it had been building silently, just as his own had.

By season's end, Marcus had played more minutes than any other midfielder on the team. No injuries. No setbacks. Just consistency. The AI system hadn't changed who he was as an athlete. It had simply shown him what his body couldn't say out loud. For the first time in his career, Marcus understood that durability wasn't about toughness alone. It was about awareness. And the greatest advantage he had wasn't strength or speed—it was knowing when to listen before the pain ever arrived.

Chapter 2

The Data Beneath the Breakdown

Every athletic injury leaves a trail long before pain appears. Muscles tighten, movement compensations emerge, recovery efficiency declines, and the nervous system begins to struggle under cumulative load. For decades, these early signals went unnoticed because they were too subtle, too complex, or too fragmented for human observation. Artificial intelligence changes this reality by turning raw athletic data into meaningful insight, revealing the hidden patterns that precede physical breakdown.

At the foundation of AI-driven injury prediction is continuous data collection. Modern athletes generate data during nearly every moment of training, competition, rest, and recovery. Wearable sensors capture heart rate variability, sleep cycles, movement acceleration, and impact forces. Cameras and motion capture systems record joint angles, stride mechanics, and force application. Training logs document workload, intensity, and volume. Even subjective inputs—such as perceived exertion, mood, and stress—become valuable data points. AI systems do not prioritize one metric over another; instead, they analyze how all metrics interact over time. One of the most important distinctions AI makes is between normal fatigue and dangerous fatigue. Fatigue is not inherently harmful; it is a necessary stimulus for adaptation. However, when fatigue accumulates faster than recovery, injury risk increases exponentially. AI evaluates this balance by analyzing trends rather than isolated values. A single poor night of sleep may not raise concern, but a gradual decline in sleep quality combined with elevated resting heart rate and reduced neuromuscular efficiency forms a recognizable risk pattern. AI excels at detecting these converging signals.

Movement data plays a central role in uncovering injury precursors. Small biomechanical changes often appear long before structural damage occurs. An athlete may subconsciously shift load away from a fatigued muscle, altering joint mechanics by fractions of a degree. Over thousands of repetitions, these micro-adjustments amplify stress on vulnerable tissues. AI systems detect these changes through precise motion tracking and compare them against the athlete's historical movement baseline. Deviations that appear insignificant to the naked eye become powerful predictors when viewed through a data-driven lens.

AI also contextualizes data based on sport-specific demands. Injury risk in a sprinter differs fundamentally from that of a swimmer, basketball player, or endurance runner. AI models are trained on sport-specific datasets that account for typical movement patterns, force demands, and injury profiles unique to each discipline. This contextual intelligence prevents false alarms and ensures predictions are relevant to the athlete's actual performance environment.

Historical data significantly enhances predictive accuracy. AI systems analyze past injuries, training loads, recovery timelines, and return-to-play outcomes to refine future predictions. An athlete with a prior hamstring strain, for example, may exhibit different risk thresholds than an athlete with no injury history. AI incorporates this history dynamically, adjusting sensitivity levels and intervention recommendations accordingly. This individualized learning process transforms injury prevention from a generalized framework into a personalized safeguard.

Another critical advantage of AI lies in temporal pattern recognition. Injuries rarely occur suddenly; they evolve through phases of increasing vulnerability. AI identifies these phases by monitoring how variables change relative to one another over time. A spike in workload may be safe if recovery metrics remain stable, but dangerous if recovery lags behind. AI recognizes not only what changes, but when it changes and in what sequence, allowing it to anticipate the tipping point before injury occurs. Psychophysiological data adds an additional layer of depth to AI analysis. Mental stress alters motor control, reaction timing, and muscle activation patterns. AI systems integrate psychological assessments, cognitive load indicators, and nervous system metrics to identify when mental fatigue may increase physical injury risk. This integration reinforces the understanding that injuries are not purely mechanical events, but systemic failures involving both mind and body.

As data accumulates, AI systems become increasingly accurate and efficient. Machine learning algorithms refine prediction models by continuously validating outcomes against real-world results. False positives are reduced, true positives become more precise, and intervention strategies become more targeted. Over time, AI transitions from a monitoring tool into an intelligent advisor—one that understands the athlete's unique physiology better with every session.

Ultimately, the power of AI injury prediction lies not in any single dataset, but in the synthesis of many. By transforming fragmented data into a coherent narrative of physical readiness, AI reveals the unseen forces shaping injury risk. This chapter demonstrates that injuries are not mysterious events; they are predictable outcomes of identifiable patterns. With the right data and intelligent analysis, breakdown becomes something that can be anticipated—and avoided.

Patterns No One Else Could See

Lena prided herself on discipline. As a collegiate long-distance runner, she tracked every mile, every split, every workout. She knew her body well—or at least she thought she did. When her program introduced AI-driven injury monitoring, Lena assumed it would simply confirm what she already knew: she was fit, consistent, and resilient.

The system quietly collected data as Lena trained. Her watch logged heart rate and pace. Cameras analyzed her stride during track workouts. Recovery surveys tracked sleep quality and perceived fatigue. Lena didn't feel different. Her times were strong. Her motivation was high. On the surface, everything looked perfect.

Halfway through the season, the AI system flagged Lena's profile for review. The alert didn't claim she was injured. Instead, it identified an emerging risk pattern associated with tibial stress injuries. The coaching staff was surprised. Lena had never missed a practice. She reported no pain. But the data showed something else.

Her stride length had shortened slightly during fatigue. Ground contact time increased during longer runs. Recovery metrics showed slower nervous system rebound after hard workouts. Sleep disruptions appeared after high-mileage weeks. Individually, each metric seemed harmless. Together, they formed a pattern Lena couldn't see—but the AI could.

When her coach suggested reducing mileage temporarily, Lena felt frustrated. She worried about losing fitness and falling behind her competitors. But the medical staff explained the trend. They showed her visual comparisons between her current movement patterns and her baseline from earlier in the season. The difference was subtle—but undeniable.

Reluctantly, Lena adjusted her training. Mileage dipped slightly. Strength work targeted the asymmetries the AI identified. Recovery protocols became non-negotiable. Weeks passed, and Lena noticed something unexpected. Her legs felt fresher late in workouts. Her pace stabilized. The heaviness she had learned to ignore faded.

Later that season, a teammate with similar training habits but no AI intervention suffered a stress fracture. Watching the season slip away for someone so dedicated shook Lena deeply. She realized how close she might have been to the same fate.

By the championship meet, Lena felt strong and confident. She ran with freedom instead of fear. When she crossed the finish line with a personal best, she understood the role the AI had played. It hadn't limited her—it had protected her from her own blind spots. Looking back, Lena realized the data hadn't changed her destiny by chance. It changed it by revealing patterns no one else could see. And in that visibility, she found the longevity every athlete hopes for but few achieve.

Chapter 3

Predictive Modeling — How AI Forecasts Injuries Before They Happen

Predicting athletic injuries requires more than identifying risk factors; it requires understanding how those factors interact over time to produce failure. Artificial intelligence accomplishes this through predictive modeling, a process in which machine learning algorithms analyze historical and real-time data to forecast future injury probability. Unlike traditional screening tools that rely on static checklists or single-variable thresholds, AI models operate dynamically, continuously recalculating risk as conditions change. This allows injury prevention strategies to shift from reactive observation to forward-looking intervention.

Predictive modeling begins with training data. AI systems are exposed to large datasets containing thousands or millions of athlete profiles, including training loads, biomechanical metrics, recovery indicators, psychological stress levels, injury histories, and return-to-play outcomes. Each dataset contains examples of both healthy performance and injury events. By analyzing these patterns, AI learns which combinations of variables most frequently precede specific injuries. This learning process is not linear; it involves recognizing complex, nonlinear relationships that human analysis cannot reliably detect.

One of the defining strengths of AI predictive models is their ability to account for time-dependent variables. Injury risk is rarely determined by a single moment; it accumulates across days, weeks, and months. AI tracks trends such as increasing workload density, declining recovery efficiency, and gradual biomechanical drift. These temporal patterns reveal vulnerability windows—periods during which the athlete is statistically more likely to experience injury. By identifying these windows early, AI enables preemptive adjustments that disrupt the progression toward breakdown.

Machine learning algorithms continuously refine predictions by comparing forecasts against real-world outcomes. When an injury occurs, the system evaluates which variables contributed most strongly to the event. When an injury is avoided, the system analyzes which interventions were effective. This feedback loop improves prediction accuracy over time, making AI models increasingly personalized. Two athletes may display similar workloads yet face different injury risks based on genetics, injury history, movement efficiency, and recovery capacity. AI adapts to these differences rather than applying uniform standards. Risk scoring is a central output of predictive modeling. AI systems translate complex datasets into interpretable risk metrics that coaches and medical staff can act upon. These scores are not binary judgments but probabilistic estimates that reflect uncertainty and confidence intervals. A rising risk score does not mean injury is inevitable; it signals that the probability of injury has increased relative to baseline. This nuanced interpretation allows decision-makers to intervene strategically rather than overreacting to isolated fluctuations.

AI predictive models also distinguish between short-term and long-term risk. Acute risk may increase rapidly due to sudden workload spikes or poor recovery, while chronic risk builds slowly through repetitive stress and unresolved compensations. AI tracks both timelines simultaneously, providing layered insights into immediate vulnerability and long-term durability. This dual perspective helps athletes manage season-long performance while safeguarding career longevity.

Another key advantage of predictive modeling is its ability to simulate alternative outcomes. AI systems can evaluate hypothetical scenarios, such as increased training volume, altered recovery schedules, or modified biomechanics, and estimate how each change affects injury risk. This allows coaches and athletes to test strategies virtually before implementing them physically. Predictive simulation transforms injury prevention into a proactive planning process rather than a reactive response.

Interpretability remains a critical consideration in AI sports medicine. Modern predictive models increasingly emphasize explainability, showing which variables contribute most to risk predictions. This transparency builds trust and encourages athlete buy-in. When athletes understand why risk is rising—whether due to sleep deficits, mechanical inefficiencies, or psychological stress—they are more likely to engage with corrective strategies. AI becomes a collaborative partner rather than a black-box authority.

As predictive modeling continues to evolve, its integration into daily training environments becomes seamless. Risk forecasts update automatically as new data arrives, providing real-time insight without disrupting workflow. This continuous intelligence allows athletes to train aggressively when conditions are favorable and adjust when vulnerability increases. The result is not reduced performance, but sustained performance across longer timelines.

Predictive modeling represents the core intelligence behind AI injury prevention. It transforms raw data into foresight, uncertainty into probability, and risk into opportunity for intervention. By forecasting injuries before they happen, AI empowers athletes to protect their bodies without compromising ambition. This chapter establishes predictive modeling as the engine that drives the future of intelligent sports medicine.

The Season That Never Broke Him

Daniel had always played on the edge. As a professional basketball guard, his style was explosive—hard cuts, aggressive drives, relentless defense. It thrilled fans but worried trainers. Every season, Daniel dealt with ankle sprains, knee inflammation, or lingering tendon pain. Injuries weren't catastrophic, but they were constant. He accepted them as the price of intensity.

When his team introduced an AI-based injury prediction system, Daniel assumed it would restrict his game. He feared being told to rest when he felt fine or being benched due to a number on a screen. But the coaching staff assured him the system wasn't about limitation—it was about longevity.

As the season began, the AI quietly monitored Daniel's workload. Practice intensity, game minutes, movement efficiency, sleep patterns, and recovery markers all fed into predictive models. Early on, everything looked stable. Daniel played freely, trusting his instincts. Midway through the season, the AI system flagged an upcoming risk window. The model predicted a high probability of knee tendinopathy within the next four weeks if Daniel's usage remained unchanged. The forecast wasn't based on pain—Daniel felt none. It was based on cumulative load patterns, subtle changes in landing mechanics, and delayed recovery after back-to-back games.

The coaching staff showed Daniel the projection. They explained how the model had identified similar patterns in past seasons—both his own and those of other players. For the first time, Daniel saw injury risk as a timeline, not a surprise. He agreed to test the plan.

Instead of reducing his competitiveness, the adjustments were surgical. His minutes were redistributed. Certain high-impact drills were replaced with low-load skill work. Recovery protocols targeted specific stress markers. The AI recalculated risk daily, adapting as Daniel responded.

Weeks passed. The predicted injury window came and went—without injury. Daniel felt stronger late in games. His explosiveness remained intact, but the nagging pain he had grown accustomed to never arrived. The AI model adjusted again, lowering his risk score as recovery stabilized.

By playoff time, Daniel was playing his best basketball. While others battled fatigue and soreness, he felt durable. Watching teammates manage injuries reinforced what he had learned: injury wasn't just bad luck. It was often a predictable outcome that could be avoided.

At the end of the season, Daniel reviewed his data with the medical staff. The AI had accurately predicted multiple high-risk periods and guided interventions that prevented breakdown. For the first time in his career, he finished a season healthy.

Daniel realized something profound. Playing on the edge didn't require sacrificing the future. With predictive intelligence guiding his path, he could compete fiercely without breaking. The season that never broke him became the standard he refused to leave behind.

Chapter 4

Intervention Intelligence — Turning Risk Forecasts Into Action

Predicting injury risk is only valuable if it leads to effective action. Artificial intelligence reaches its true potential in sports medicine when predictive insights are transformed into timely, intelligent interventions. Once AI systems identify rising injury probability, they guide decisions that adjust training, recovery, movement patterns, and competition exposure. This process replaces reactive guesswork with structured, data-driven responses that protect the athlete without sacrificing performance.

AI-guided intervention begins with prioritization. Not all risk signals require the same response. Some indicate immediate danger, while others suggest long-term vulnerability. AI evaluates the severity, trajectory, and confidence level of each prediction before recommending action. A rapidly rising acute risk score may trigger immediate workload reduction, while a slow-building chronic risk may prompt gradual biomechanical corrections or recovery enhancements. This prioritization ensures interventions are proportional rather than disruptive. Training load modulation is one of the most common AI-driven interventions. When injury risk increases, AI systems assess which components of training contribute most to overload. Instead of reducing overall training indiscriminately, AI targets specific stressors such as high-impact drills, excessive volume density, or repeated maximal efforts. This precision allows athletes to maintain skill development and conditioning while reducing tissue strain. Load adjustments become surgical rather than blunt.

Recovery optimization is another critical intervention pathway. AI evaluates recovery markers including heart rate variability, sleep quality, nervous system readiness, and subjective fatigue. When recovery lags behind workload, AI recommends targeted recovery strategies such as altered training schedules, enhanced sleep protocols, or low-intensity movement sessions. These recommendations are individualized, recognizing that recovery capacity varies widely between athletes and fluctuates across seasons.

Biomechanical intervention plays a vital role in injury prevention. When AI detects movement inefficiencies or compensatory patterns, it links these findings to corrective strategies. This may involve targeted strength exercises, mobility work, neuromuscular re-education, or technique adjustments. AI continuously monitors whether interventions improve movement quality, ensuring corrections are effective rather than theoretical. This feedback loop accelerates adaptation and reduces reinjury risk.

AI also supports decision-making around competition exposure. In high-stakes environments, athletes are often asked to perform despite elevated risk. AI provides objective insight into how much risk is increasing and what trade-offs exist. Coaches and medical staff use this information to make informed decisions about minutes played, positional assignments, or substitution timing. Rather than relying on emotion or pressure, decisions are grounded in probability and data.

Psychological intervention is an often-overlooked aspect of AI-guided injury prevention. When mental stress contributes to physical vulnerability, AI systems flag this connection and recommend appropriate responses. These may include reduced cognitive load, altered practice structure, mindfulness strategies, or communication adjustments. By addressing psychological stress alongside physical strain, AI ensures interventions support the athlete as a whole.

One of the most powerful features of AI intervention systems is adaptability. Interventions are not fixed prescriptions; they evolve based on athlete response. If risk decreases after adjustments, AI gradually restores training intensity. If risk persists, strategies are refined. This continuous calibration ensures athletes remain challenged without crossing into danger. Intervention becomes a dynamic process rather than a one-time correction.

Trust is essential for successful AI-guided intervention. Athletes are more likely to follow recommendations when they understand the rationale behind them. Modern AI systems emphasize transparency, explaining which factors contributed most to risk and how proposed interventions address those factors. This clarity transforms AI from an external authority into a collaborative partner, strengthening athlete buy-in and compliance.

At scale, AI-guided intervention reshapes sports medicine culture. Injury prevention becomes proactive, personalized, and integrated into daily training rather than isolated in medical departments. Athletes train with greater confidence, knowing interventions are based on objective insight rather than intuition alone. The result is not cautious performance, but sustainable excellence built on intelligent decision-making.

This chapter demonstrates that AI injury prediction is only the first step. The true power lies in how that knowledge is applied. When forecasts guide action with precision and adaptability, AI becomes the bridge between awareness and durability—protecting athletes while allowing them to compete at their highest level.

The Choice That Saved the Season

Ryan was having the best year of his career. As a professional hockey forward, he felt fast, strong, and confident. His minutes were climbing, his scoring was consistent, and his name was circulating in award conversations. When the AI injury monitoring system flagged elevated hip and groin risk, Ryan dismissed it immediately. He felt unstoppable.

The coaching staff reviewed the data carefully. The AI model showed a steady rise in cumulative load, declining recovery markers, and subtle changes in skating mechanics during high-speed transitions. The system projected a significant probability of groin strain within the next three weeks if no adjustments were made. Ryan didn't feel pain, but the numbers told a story he couldn't feel yet.

The proposed intervention wasn't dramatic. Slightly reduced practice volume. Targeted mobility and neuromuscular work. Adjusted shift lengths during games. Ryan hesitated. The season was peaking, and he didn't want anything to interrupt his momentum. But after a long conversation with the medical team, he agreed to trust the process. The changes felt strange at first. Shorter practices. More emphasis on recovery. Focused corrective drills instead of endless repetitions. Ryan worried it would dull his edge. Instead, he noticed his legs felt fresher late in games. His acceleration improved. The tightness he had learned to ignore slowly disappeared.

Two weeks later, a teammate playing through similar workload patterns suffered a groin tear that ended his season. Watching from the bench, Ryan felt a knot in his stomach. He realized how close he might have been to the same outcome. The AI alert hadn't been an inconvenience—it had been a warning.

As the playoffs approached, Ryan's risk score dropped steadily. The AI system gradually increased his workload, matching his improved recovery and mechanics. By postseason play, Ryan was at full intensity without the underlying vulnerability that once shadowed him.

Ryan finished the season healthy, productive, and proud—not because he pushed through risk, but because he respected it. The choice to intervene early didn't limit his performance. It preserved it. The season that could have ended abruptly became the season that defined his career.

When asked later what changed, Ryan didn't credit luck or toughness. He credited awareness. He learned that the smartest athletes aren't the ones who ignore risk—but the ones who act on it before it acts on them.

Chapter 5

AI Rehabilitation & Return-to-Play Intelligence

Injury prevention does not end when an athlete gets hurt. In many cases, the greatest risk occurs during rehabilitation and return to play, when incomplete healing, compensation patterns, or rushed timelines lead to reinjury. Artificial intelligence fundamentally reshapes rehabilitation by replacing time-based recovery assumptions with data-driven readiness assessments. Instead of asking how long an injury should take to heal, AI asks whether the athlete's body is actually prepared to perform again.

Traditional rehabilitation protocols often rely on generalized timelines and subjective evaluations. While these approaches can be effective, they fail to account for individual variability in healing, neuromuscular control, and psychological readiness. AI-driven rehabilitation systems monitor objective markers such as movement symmetry, force production, coordination timing, tissue loading tolerance, and nervous system recovery. These systems provide continuous insight into how the athlete is responding to rehabilitation stress, ensuring progress without premature exposure to risk. A key advantage of AI in rehabilitation is its ability to identify compensatory movement patterns. After injury, athletes frequently shift load away from the injured area, even when pain subsides. These compensations may protect the injured tissue temporarily but increase stress elsewhere, setting the stage for secondary injuries. AI systems detect these subtle changes through motion capture, force analysis, and neuromuscular timing data, allowing clinicians to correct them before they become ingrained habits.

AI also enhances exercise progression within rehabilitation programs. Rather than advancing exercises based solely on time or repetition counts, AI evaluates performance quality and physiological response. If an athlete demonstrates sufficient control, strength, and recovery capacity, progression accelerates. If fatigue, asymmetry, or instability emerges, progression slows. This adaptive approach ensures rehabilitation remains challenging without exceeding tissue tolerance.

Psychological readiness is a critical but often underestimated component of return-to-play decisions. Fear of reinjury alters movement patterns, reaction time, and decision-making under pressure. AI systems integrate psychological assessments, stress markers, and behavioral data to evaluate mental readiness alongside physical recovery. By addressing psychological barriers early, AI helps athletes regain confidence and fluidity, reducing reinjury risk caused by hesitation or overprotection.

Return-to-play decisions benefit greatly from AI-driven probability modeling. Rather than issuing binary clearance decisions, AI provides risk estimates that reflect uncertainty and context. These models consider sport demands, position-specific loads, competition intensity, and recent workload exposure. This allows medical teams to design graduated return strategies, easing athletes back into competition rather than forcing abrupt transitions from rehabilitation to full performance.

AI systems also support post-return monitoring. Injury risk does not disappear once an athlete resumes competition; it often remains elevated during the initial weeks back. AI continues to track recovery markers, workload tolerance, and movement quality, adjusting training and competition exposure as needed. This extended oversight reduces reinjury rates and supports long-term durability rather than short-term clearance.

Collaboration remains central to AI-powered rehabilitation. The most effective systems integrate input from physical therapists, athletic trainers, physicians, coaches, and athletes. AI does not replace clinical expertise; it enhances it by providing objective, continuous insight. When combined with human judgment, AI enables rehabilitation strategies that are both precise and compassionate.

Ultimately, AI transforms rehabilitation from a waiting process into an active optimization phase. Injuries become opportunities to rebuild movement efficiency, address underlying weaknesses, and improve resilience. By guiding athletes through intelligent rehabilitation and safe return-to-play decisions, AI completes the injury prevention cycle—protecting not just the present season, but the athlete's long-term career.

Cleared When the Body Was Ready

Sophia had torn her ACL before. The first time, recovery was defined by a calendar. Six months post-surgery, she returned to competition because the timeline said she could. Three weeks later, she reinjured the same knee. The second injury hurt more emotionally than physically. She began to doubt whether her body would ever feel trustworthy again.

After her second surgery, Sophia joined a training facility that used AI-driven rehabilitation systems. This time, recovery didn't revolve around dates on a chart. Sensors tracked her movement daily. Cameras analyzed her landing mechanics. Force plates measured how evenly she distributed load through her legs. The AI system quietly built a profile of her recovery—one data point at a time.

Early on, Sophia felt strong, but the AI showed lingering asymmetries. Her injured leg avoided full load during deceleration. Neuromuscular timing lagged slightly under fatigue. She felt discouraged, but the therapists explained that this insight was protection, not failure. The system adjusted her program, emphasizing control and confidence rather than speed.

Weeks passed, and the data began to change. Symmetry improved. Reaction timing normalized. Recovery scores stabilized even as training intensity increased. The AI system recalculated her return-to-play risk continuously, showing steady improvement rather than a fixed endpoint.

When Sophia finally returned to team practice, it wasn't because a calendar allowed it—it was because her body demonstrated readiness. Even then, the AI recommended controlled exposure: limited minutes, gradual increases, constant monitoring. Sophia felt supported rather than rushed.

Her first game back was emotional. Every cut and jump carried memory, but not fear. She moved freely, trusting her knee instead of bracing against it. As the season progressed,

Sophia grew stronger than she had been before the injury—not just physically, but mentally.

By season's end, Sophia had played every match without setback. Reviewing her recovery data, she saw something powerful. The AI system didn't just return her to play—it rebuilt her confidence. For the first time, clearance meant readiness, not risk.

Sophia learned that healing wasn't about time passing. It was about signals aligning. And when those signals finally said "go," she knew it was true.

Chapter 6

Ethics, Data Privacy & Athlete Autonomy in AI Sports Medicine

As artificial intelligence becomes more deeply integrated into sports medicine, ethical considerations move from the margins to the center of athletic decision-making. AI systems collect, analyze, and interpret intimate biological, behavioral, and psychological data. While this information enables unprecedented injury prevention and performance optimization, it also raises critical questions about privacy, consent, ownership, and control. Ethical implementation determines whether AI becomes an empowering ally or a source of exploitation within sports environments.

Data privacy is one of the most pressing concerns in AI-driven sports medicine. Athletes generate sensitive data related to health status, injury risk, mental stress, recovery capacity, and long-term durability. If mishandled, this data can influence contract negotiations, playing time, selection decisions, or public perception. Ethical AI systems prioritize secure data storage, encryption, limited access, and strict usage policies. Athletes must be confident that their data is protected and used solely for their well-being rather than organizational advantage. Informed consent is fundamental to ethical AI use.

Athletes should understand what data is collected, how it is analyzed, and how conclusions are applied. Consent should be ongoing rather than a one-time agreement, allowing athletes to revisit participation as systems evolve. Transparent communication builds trust and ensures athletes remain active participants rather than passive data sources. Without informed consent, even well-intentioned AI systems risk undermining athlete autonomy.

Ownership of data is another critical ethical dimension. Athletes increasingly question who controls the information generated by their bodies. Ethical frameworks recognize athletes as primary data owners, granting them access, portability, and authority over how their data is shared. Teams and organizations function as stewards rather than owners, using data collaboratively to support athlete health. This shift in perspective rebalances power dynamics and reinforces athlete-centered care.

Bias within AI models presents additional ethical challenges. If training datasets lack diversity across gender, age, ethnicity, or sport, predictions may be less accurate or even harmful for underrepresented groups. Ethical AI development requires inclusive datasets and continuous auditing to identify and correct bias. Systems must adapt to individual variability rather than forcing athletes into generalized norms that may not reflect their physiology or context.

Athlete autonomy must remain central to AI-guided decision-making. AI systems provide recommendations, not mandates. Final decisions should involve dialogue between athletes, medical professionals, and coaches. When AI overrides athlete input or becomes a tool for coercion, its value erodes. Ethical implementation empowers athletes with information, enabling informed choices rather than enforcing compliance.

Transparency strengthens ethical trust. Athletes are more likely to embrace AI systems when they understand why risk scores rise, how predictions are generated, and what factors influence recommendations. Explainable AI transforms complex models into understandable insights, demystifying technology and fostering collaboration. When athletes see AI as a partner rather than a judge, adherence improves and resistance declines.

The ethical use of AI also extends to competitive fairness. Access to advanced AI systems may create disparities between well-funded programs and under-resourced athletes. As technology becomes more widespread, ethical adoption includes efforts to democratize access and prevent the creation of unequal playing fields. Injury prevention should not become a privilege reserved for the elite. Long-term data stewardship represents a final ethical consideration. AI systems often retain historical data to improve predictions over time. Ethical policies define how long data is stored, when it is anonymized, and how it is used after an athlete retires. Respecting athletes beyond their competitive years reinforces trust and ensures AI systems contribute positively across the entire athletic lifespan.

Ethical AI in sports medicine is not an obstacle to progress; it is a prerequisite for sustainable innovation. When privacy, autonomy, and transparency are prioritized, AI strengthens rather than threatens athlete welfare. This chapter underscores that the future of injury prevention depends not only on technological capability, but on ethical responsibility.

More Than a Data Point

Jamal had always trusted his instincts. As a professional football player, he relied on feel—how his body responded, how his mind reacted under pressure. When his team introduced an advanced AI injury prediction system, Jamal felt uneasy. The technology promised protection, but he worried it would become a silent judge determining his future.

During preseason, Jamal learned that the system tracked everything: workload, sleep, movement efficiency, stress levels. When his risk score rose after a series of intense practices, the coaching staff discussed reducing his reps. Jamal felt blindsided. No one had explained how the system worked or why the number mattered.

Instead of pushing back, Jamal asked questions. The medical team sat down with him and walked through the data. They showed how accumulated fatigue, reduced recovery, and subtle movement changes had contributed to the elevated risk score. They explained what the system could—and could not—decide. Jamal realized the AI wasn't making choices for him; it was offering insight he didn't have before.

As the season progressed, Jamal became more involved in the process. He reviewed his data regularly, learned which factors influenced his risk, and communicated openly about how he felt physically and mentally. When recommendations aligned with his own instincts, trust grew. When they didn't, discussions followed. Decisions became collaborative rather than imposed.

One week, Jamal's risk score spiked again. This time, he wasn't alarmed. He recognized the pattern—poor sleep after travel, high cognitive stress, increased workload. He chose to adjust his routine proactively, prioritizing recovery and communication. The risk score dropped within days.

Late in the season, a teammate resisted the system entirely, dismissing its warnings as interference. He played through mounting risk and suffered a significant injury that sidelined him indefinitely. Watching from the sidelines, Jamal reflected on the difference. The technology hadn't failed his teammate—trust had.

By season's end, Jamal finished healthy, productive, and confident. The AI system never replaced his judgment; it sharpened it. He realized that ethical technology didn't take control away—it gave him clarity.

Jamal learned that he was never just a data point. When used responsibly, AI didn't define him. It respected him. And that respect made all the difference.

Chapter 7

Protecting Athletes for Life — Youth, Amateur & Aging Populations

Athletic injury prevention must extend beyond elite professionals to protect athletes at every stage of life. Youth athletes, recreational competitors, collegiate players, and aging athletes all face unique injury risks shaped by growth, lifestyle demands, and physiological change. Artificial intelligence offers a unified framework capable of adapting injury prevention strategies across these diverse populations, ensuring that safety, development, and longevity remain central regardless of performance level.

Youth athletes are among the most vulnerable populations due to rapid physical growth, immature neuromuscular control, and increasing training specialization at younger ages. Growth spurts alter limb length, coordination, and force absorption patterns, increasing injury risk if training loads remain unchanged. AI systems monitor movement variability, workload tolerance, and recovery capacity during developmental phases, identifying periods when athletes are particularly vulnerable. This allows coaches and parents to adjust training proactively rather than reacting to overuse injuries after they occur.

Overuse injuries are especially prevalent among youth and adolescent athletes due to early sport specialization and year-round competition. AI excels at tracking cumulative load across practices, games, and informal play, providing a holistic picture of total stress exposure. By identifying excessive repetition or insufficient recovery, AI helps prevent stress fractures, tendon injuries, and joint damage that can have lifelong consequences. This data-driven oversight supports healthy development rather than premature burnout.

Amateur and recreational athletes face a different set of challenges. Balancing training with work, family, and inconsistent schedules often leads to irregular recovery and sudden workload spikes. Weekend competitions, travel, and stress outside sport increase injury risk despite lower overall training volume. AI systems integrate lifestyle data such as sleep disruption, stress indicators, and irregular training patterns to predict injury risk more accurately in non-professional populations. This personalized insight empowers athletes to train intelligently without sacrificing health.

Collegiate athletes occupy a unique middle ground between youth development and professional performance. Academic stress, travel demands, and compressed competition schedules create complex risk environments. AI helps manage these pressures by identifying when cognitive load and physical stress converge, increasing injury vulnerability. By providing objective insight, AI supports better communication between athletes, coaches, and medical staff, reducing pressure-driven decisions that compromise long-term well-being.

Aging athletes represent another critical population where AI injury prevention delivers immense value. As connective tissue elasticity decreases, recovery slows, and injury tolerance narrows with age. AI systems adjust expectations and recommendations based on age-related physiological changes, ensuring training remains effective without exceeding tissue capacity. By identifying subtle declines in recovery efficiency or movement stability, AI helps older athletes maintain performance safely rather than retreating from competition prematurely.

AI also plays a powerful role in preserving lifelong athletic participation. Many individuals disengage from sport after repeated injuries or chronic pain. By preventing avoidable breakdowns, AI enables athletes to remain active longer, supporting physical health, mental well-being, and social connection. Injury prevention becomes a public health benefit rather than a performance luxury.

Education is a vital component of AI adoption across non-elite populations. When athletes understand why recommendations exist, compliance improves. AI systems increasingly provide clear explanations and visual feedback tailored to non-technical users. This transparency empowers athletes, parents, and coaches to make informed decisions without fear or confusion.

Equity and accessibility remain important considerations. Ethical deployment of AI in youth and amateur settings emphasizes affordability, simplicity, and privacy protection. As technology evolves, scalable solutions ensure that injury prevention benefits are not limited to elite programs. Protecting athletes for life requires expanding access rather than concentrating advantage.

Ultimately, AI reframes athletic success as durability across decades rather than peaks measured in seasons. By adapting injury prediction and prevention strategies to each stage of life, AI ensures athletes are protected not only during competition, but throughout their lifelong relationship with sport. This chapter highlights AI's role in creating healthier athletic ecosystems where performance and longevity coexist.

Still in the Game

Ethan was twelve when he first tore his shoulder. A promising baseball pitcher, he had been playing year-round since age eight. His parents trusted coaches who said pain was normal and rest was optional. By high school, Ethan's shoulder hurt more often than it didn't. Doctors warned him his future in the sport was uncertain.

Years later, Ethan returned to baseball as a recreational adult player. This time, things were different. His league partnered with a sports science clinic using AI-driven injury monitoring. Ethan was skeptical at first, but he agreed to participate. The system tracked his throwing volume, recovery, sleep, and movement efficiency. For the first time, someone was watching the whole picture.

Early data revealed what Ethan had always suspected. His shoulder compensated during fatigue, increasing stress on vulnerable tissues. The AI system recommended specific rest intervals and minor mechanical adjustments. More importantly, it showed him why those changes mattered.

As the season progressed, Ethan stayed healthy. He felt stronger—not because he pushed harder, but because he trained smarter. Watching younger players struggle with injuries reminded him of his own early years. He encouraged them to listen when the data spoke.

Meanwhile, Ethan's father joined the league too. In his fifties, he had assumed competitive sports were behind him. The AI system adjusted recommendations based on age, recovery capacity, and prior injuries. Together, father and son trained safely, sharing a connection through sport that had nearly been lost.

By season's end, Ethan realized something profound. AI hadn't changed his love for the game—it had preserved it. He wasn't chasing records anymore. He was chasing moments, health, and longevity.

Standing on the field one evening, Ethan looked around at players of all ages. Some were young and dreaming big. Others were older and just grateful to be moving. AI had given them all the same gift: the chance to stay in the game longer than they ever thought possible.

And for Ethan, that was the greatest win of all.

Chapter 8

Scaling Intelligence — Team, Program & Organizational Implementation

Artificial intelligence delivers its greatest impact when injury prevention is embedded not only at the individual level, but across entire teams, programs, and organizations. While personalized insights protect individual athletes, organizational implementation ensures consistency, sustainability, and cultural alignment. AI-driven sports medicine transforms from a tool into an ecosystem when it informs coaching strategy, medical workflows, training design, and leadership decisions simultaneously.

Team-wide AI implementation begins with data standardization. Inconsistent data collection undermines predictive accuracy and trust. Successful programs establish uniform protocols for wearable usage, movement capture, recovery assessments, and subjective reporting. These protocols are designed to integrate seamlessly into daily routines, minimizing disruption while maximizing data quality. Consistency allows AI systems to compare athletes accurately, identify team-wide risk trends, and optimize training loads collectively rather than reactively. Communication architecture is critical when scaling AI systems. Injury risk insights must flow clearly between medical staff, coaches, performance specialists, and athletes. AI platforms increasingly translate complex analytics into intuitive dashboards tailored to each role. Coaches view workload readiness and availability forecasts. Medical teams access detailed biomechanical and recovery metrics. Athletes receive simplified insights focused on action rather than analysis. This role-based communication prevents information overload while preserving transparency.

Organizational trust determines whether AI systems are embraced or resisted. Athletes and coaches must believe that AI insights serve health and performance rather than surveillance or control. Leadership sets this tone by defining ethical boundaries, clarifying data usage policies, and reinforcing athlete-first decision-making. When AI is positioned as a protective system rather than an evaluative weapon, adoption accelerates and resistance declines.

Training periodization benefits significantly from team-level AI insights. By analyzing cumulative stress across the roster, AI identifies optimal windows for high-intensity training, recovery emphasis, or tactical focus. Rather than pushing all athletes through identical schedules, teams adapt workloads dynamically based on readiness profiles. This reduces collective fatigue and minimizes injury clusters that often emerge during congested competition periods. AI also supports strategic roster management. Availability forecasting allows organizations to anticipate potential absences weeks in advance, enabling proactive rotation planning rather than emergency adjustments. Medical and performance teams collaborate with coaching staff to balance competitiveness with durability. Over time, this reduces injury-related volatility and improves season-long consistency.

Integration with existing medical infrastructure is essential for successful scaling. AI systems complement rather than replace clinical expertise. Physical therapists, athletic trainers, and physicians contribute qualitative insights that enhance model accuracy. Feedback loops between human expertise and AI analytics refine predictions and interventions continuously. This hybrid approach strengthens outcomes while preserving professional judgment.

Education and onboarding play a vital role in organization-wide adoption. Athletes and staff must understand how AI systems work, what they measure, and how recommendations are generated. Training sessions, ongoing feedback, and transparent reporting foster literacy and confidence. As understanding increases, compliance improves and AI becomes a trusted advisor rather than an external authority. Scalability also introduces logistical challenges. Data security, infrastructure capacity, and system maintenance require dedicated oversight. Organizations establish governance structures to manage updates, audits, and ethical compliance. Long-term success depends on treating AI injury prevention as a strategic investment rather than a temporary experiment.

Ultimately, team-wide AI implementation redefines performance culture. Success is measured not only by wins, but by availability, resilience, and sustained output. Organizations that embrace AI holistically gain a competitive advantage rooted in health intelligence. This chapter demonstrates that AI injury prevention reaches its full potential when embedded into the collective fabric of sport rather than isolated at the individual level.

The Season the Team Stayed Whole

Coach Ramirez had seen it too many times. A strong start, followed by injuries that slowly unraveled the season. Talent didn't disappear — availability did. When the organization decided to implement a team-wide AI injury prevention system, Ramirez was cautious. He worried it would complicate decisions or interfere with instincts built over decades.

The rollout began quietly. Players wore tracking devices during training. Recovery check-ins became routine. Dashboards replaced guesswork. At first, Ramirez glanced at the numbers skeptically, trusting his eyes more than graphs. But patterns emerged quickly.

Midway through preseason, the AI system flagged elevated risk across multiple starters. Instead of panicking, the staff adjusted training intensity and redistributed workload. Ramirez noticed something unexpected: performance improved. Practices felt sharper. Players finished sessions energized rather than exhausted.

As the season progressed, the AI platform highlighted subtle warning signs. A defensive unit trending toward overload. A veteran nearing recovery limits after travel. Decisions that once relied on instinct now had data-backed clarity. Ramirez didn't feel replaced — he felt supported.

One critical week, the system predicted an injury cluster if training continued unchanged. Ramirez adjusted rotations and emphasized recovery. Rival teams pushed hard that same week and suffered multiple injuries. His team stayed healthy.

By playoff time, something remarkable had happened. The roster was intact. Players trusted the system because it had proven itself. Communication improved. Blame disappeared. Decisions felt collective rather than imposed.

After the final match, Ramirez reviewed the season data. Injuries were down significantly. Availability was up. Performance consistency was higher than any previous year. The AI system hadn't changed the team's identity – it had protected it.

Standing in the locker room, Ramirez realized leadership had evolved. Winning wasn't about squeezing every ounce from players. It was about building systems that allowed them to give their best, week after week.

For the first time in his career, the team didn't survive the season. They mastered it – together.

Chapter 9

The Predictive Ecosystem — The Future of AI Injury Prevention

Artificial intelligence in sports medicine is evolving from isolated tools into interconnected predictive ecosystems. Early AI systems focused on single athletes, single data streams, or isolated injury risks. The next generation integrates multiple systems—wearables, biomechanics platforms, medical records, environmental data, and psychological metrics—into unified networks that continuously learn and adapt. This ecosystem approach transforms injury prevention from localized decision-making into an intelligent, anticipatory framework that spans teams, seasons, and careers.

At the core of the predictive ecosystem is interoperability. Future AI systems no longer operate in silos. Training data, medical imaging, rehabilitation progress, competition schedules, travel demands, and even environmental conditions such as temperature, altitude, and surface quality feed into shared models. By correlating these variables, AI gains deeper contextual awareness, allowing it to identify risk patterns that would otherwise remain hidden. Injury prevention becomes situational rather than generic. Networked learning dramatically accelerates prediction accuracy. When anonymized data from multiple teams, leagues, or training centers is aggregated responsibly, AI models learn from a vastly expanded dataset. Patterns that appear rare at the individual level become clear at scale. This collective intelligence allows systems to identify emerging injury trends, refine early-warning signals, and adapt faster than any single organization could independently.

Predictive ecosystems also enable cross-injury modeling. Rather than focusing on one injury type at a time, AI systems learn how different vulnerabilities interact. A slight ankle instability may increase knee injury risk. Sleep disruption may amplify muscle strain probability. Psychological stress may alter biomechanics. By understanding these interdependencies, AI shifts from linear prediction to systems-level foresight.

Real-time feedback loops are a defining feature of advanced AI ecosystems. Data updates continuously during training, competition, and recovery. AI models recalculate risk dynamically, adjusting recommendations as conditions change. This real-time intelligence allows organizations to respond immediately to emerging threats rather than relying on retrospective analysis. Injury prevention becomes a living process rather than a static plan. Environmental intelligence plays an increasing role in predictive ecosystems. Travel schedules, time zone changes, climate conditions, and playing surfaces influence injury risk more than previously acknowledged. AI integrates these variables into forecasts, helping teams plan training intensity, recovery emphasis, and rotation strategies around external stressors. Contextual awareness enhances decision quality without increasing complexity for end users.

Digital twins represent one of the most advanced applications of AI injury ecosystems. These virtual representations of individual athletes simulate how bodies respond to different training loads, recovery strategies, and competition demands. By testing scenarios in a digital environment, coaches and medical staff explore potential outcomes without physical risk. Digital twins elevate injury prevention from prediction to simulation-based planning.

Longitudinal insight is another major advantage of predictive ecosystems. AI systems track athletes across years, capturing how bodies adapt, decline, and recover over time. This historical perspective supports smarter career planning, load management, and transition strategies. Injury prevention evolves from short-term protection to long-term preservation.

Ethical governance becomes increasingly important as ecosystems grow. Shared data networks require strict safeguards to ensure privacy, consent, and equitable use. Transparent governance structures define who accesses data, how insights are applied, and how athletes remain protected within interconnected systems. Trust remains the foundation of sustainable innovation.

Ultimately, predictive ecosystems redefine sports medicine as an intelligence discipline rather than a reactive service. By connecting data, learning collectively, and anticipating risk systemically, AI moves beyond injury prevention toward resilience engineering. This chapter illustrates how the future of sports health is not about avoiding injury in isolation, but about building intelligent systems that support performance stability across entire athletic environments.

Before the Pattern Broke the League

The league didn't notice the pattern at first. Injuries always happened. That was part of the game. But by midseason, something felt different. Star players across multiple teams were sidelined with similar soft-tissue injuries. Coaches blamed scheduling. Players blamed fatigue. Medical staff treated symptoms as they appeared.

Only the AI network saw the pattern forming.

Across dozens of teams, anonymized data flowed into a shared injury prediction ecosystem. Training loads, travel schedules, recovery metrics, and biomechanical data merged silently in the background. The system detected a convergence: compressed travel, reduced sleep, and surface transitions were creating a league-wide vulnerability window.

The alert reached league officials quietly. It wasn't dramatic—just a probability curve rising faster than expected. The recommendation wasn't drastic either. Adjust scheduling intensity. Modify recovery protocols. Encourage teams to adapt workloads during specific weeks.

Some organizations listened. Others dismissed it as overreach.

Within weeks, the difference was obvious. Teams that followed the recommendations stayed relatively healthy. Teams that ignored them watched their rosters thin. Fans questioned coaching decisions. Analysts searched for explanations. The AI system simply updated its models.

One team in particular became a case study. Their staff embraced the ecosystem fully, integrating league-level insights with internal data. Coaches adjusted rotations. Medical staff emphasized recovery during high-risk windows. Players felt supported rather than restricted.

As the season progressed, injuries declined across participating teams. The league quietly expanded the system, refining governance and communication. By playoffs, availability was higher than in previous years.

Years later, the league reflected on that season as a turning point. Not because injuries disappeared—but because they became predictable at scale. The ecosystem didn't remove risk. It revealed it early enough to matter.

For the athletes, the change was subtle but powerful. Fewer surprises. More trust. Longer careers. The game remained intense—but it became smarter.

And for the AI system, the lesson was clear. Intelligence doesn't live in isolation. It thrives when patterns are shared, understood, and acted upon before they break the system they're meant to protect.

Chapter 10

Redefining Peak Performance – Durability as the New Competitive Edge

For generations, peak performance in sport has been defined by short-lived extremes: maximum speed, maximum strength, maximum output at any cost. Athletes were celebrated for pushing beyond limits, even when those limits led to breakdown. Artificial intelligence challenges this legacy by reframing peak performance as a balance between intensity and sustainability. In the AI-driven era, the most competitive athletes are not those who peak the highest for the shortest time, but those who remain available, adaptable, and resilient across longer careers.

AI injury prediction reveals a fundamental truth long ignored in sports culture: performance consistency is the greatest competitive advantage. An athlete who performs at ninety-five percent capacity for an entire season often outperforms one who reaches one hundred percent briefly before injury. By minimizing downtime, reducing reinjury cycles, and preserving readiness, AI enables athletes to express their abilities more often and more reliably. Peak performance becomes a function of durability rather than reckless output. Durability is not passive. It is an active, measurable quality shaped by biomechanics, recovery efficiency, nervous system regulation, psychological resilience, and intelligent load management. AI systems quantify these dimensions continuously, providing insight into how durability fluctuates over time. Rather than guessing when an athlete is ready to push or pull back, AI replaces intuition with evidence-based clarity. This precision allows athletes to train aggressively without crossing into destructive territory.

Longevity emerges as a natural outcome of AI-guided performance management. Athletes who avoid unnecessary injuries accumulate years of high-quality training, skill refinement, and competitive experience. AI systems track long-term adaptation trends, identifying strategies that preserve tissue health and neuromuscular efficiency across decades. This longitudinal intelligence transforms career planning from reactive survival to proactive design.

The psychological impact of durability-focused performance is profound. Athletes who trust their bodies compete with confidence rather than fear. AI reduces uncertainty by making risk visible and manageable. When athletes understand why adjustments are recommended, they engage willingly rather than resisting change. Confidence grows not from denial of risk, but from mastery over it. AI also reshapes coaching philosophy. Coaches shift from maximizing short-term output to optimizing availability and readiness. Training plans become fluid rather than rigid, adapting to real-time conditions. Success metrics expand beyond wins and losses to include injury rates, recovery stability, and roster availability. Organizations that embrace this broader definition of performance gain a sustainable edge.

Cultural transformation is perhaps AI's most lasting contribution. As data replaces mythology, toughness is redefined. Playing through pain is no longer heroic when it leads to avoidable absence. Smart restraint becomes a sign of professionalism. Athletes are empowered to listen to their bodies with the support of objective intelligence, dismantling stigma around rest and recovery.

The future of peak performance is not about creating superhuman athletes who ignore limits. It is about building intelligent systems that respect human physiology while unlocking its full potential. AI does not lower standards; it raises them by demanding consistency, accountability, and awareness. Performance excellence becomes sustainable rather than sacrificial.

This chapter concludes the journey of AI injury prediction by establishing a new paradigm. Peak performance is no longer measured by isolated moments of brilliance, but by the ability to show up—healthy, prepared, and confident—again and again. In this future, durability is not the opposite of greatness. It is the foundation of it.

The Longest Season of His Life

When Marcus entered the league, everyone talked about his ceiling. Explosive speed. Rare strength. Unstoppable potential. But by his fifth season, people talked about something else—his injuries. Hamstrings. Ankles. Back issues. Each year followed the same arc: brilliance, breakdown, recovery, repeat.

When his organization introduced AI-driven injury intelligence, Marcus was skeptical. He had heard promises before. He didn't want to be told to slow down. He wanted to be great.

The first season under the new system felt different. Marcus didn't train less—he trained smarter. The AI flagged risk windows before pain arrived. Workloads shifted subtly. Recovery became intentional rather than optional. For the first time, Marcus finished a season without missing significant time.

The second season was even better. His performance didn't spike dramatically—but it never dipped. He played nearly every game. His stats climbed steadily. Coaches trusted his availability. Teammates relied on his presence. By the third season, Marcus noticed something unexpected. Younger players were burning out. Flashing early, fading fast. Meanwhile, he felt composed. Durable. Confident. He wasn't chasing highlight moments anymore—he was building something bigger.

Late one night, reviewing his career data with the performance staff, Marcus saw the truth clearly. His best seasons weren't defined by peak outputs. They were defined by continuity. The seasons where he stayed healthy were the seasons where his impact multiplied.

Years later, when Marcus finally retired, analysts debated his legacy. He wasn't the most explosive athlete they had seen. But he was one of the most reliable. One of the most durable. One of the most consistently excellent.

Standing on the field one last time, Marcus smiled. AI hadn't made him less aggressive. It had made him wiser. He had learned that greatness wasn't about burning bright and fast—it was about staying in the game long enough to matter.

And that lesson lasted longer than any highlight ever could.

Epilogue

The Era of Intelligent Longevity

The future of sport is no longer defined by how hard an athlete can push, but by how intelligently they can endure. Throughout history, athletic greatness has often been measured in moments—record-breaking performances, championship runs, flashes of brilliance that captivate audiences and then fade. But as artificial intelligence reshapes sports medicine, training, and performance science, a new definition of greatness is emerging—one rooted in longevity, resilience, and sustained excellence.

This book has traced the evolution of injury prevention from reactive treatment to predictive intelligence. What once relied on pain signals, intuition, and delayed diagnosis has become a sophisticated system capable of detecting risk before breakdown occurs. Artificial intelligence does not remove challenge from sport. It removes unnecessary loss. It allows athletes to train hard, compete fiercely, and still protect the one asset that matters more than any stat: availability.

The most profound shift introduced by AI is not technological—it is philosophical. Athletes no longer have to choose between performance and preservation. The false trade-off between pushing limits and protecting health dissolves when risk becomes visible and manageable. With AI, restraint is no longer weakness, and rest is no longer failure. They become strategic tools in the pursuit of excellence.

Durability, once an afterthought, now stands at the center of elite performance. An athlete who remains healthy accumulates skill, experience, confidence, and tactical intelligence that short-lived peaks cannot replicate. Over time, durability compounds into dominance. AI makes this durability measurable, trainable, and repeatable, transforming it from luck into design.

This transformation extends beyond professionals. Youth athletes are protected from burnout and overuse. Amateur athletes learn to balance ambition with real-world demands. Aging athletes discover that decline is not inevitable—it is manageable. AI democratizes high-level injury prevention, making intelligent care accessible across the lifespan of sport. In doing so, it reshapes athletic participation from something people grow out of into something they can sustain.

Coaches, organizations, and institutions also evolve in this new era. Leadership shifts from extraction to optimization. Success is no longer defined solely by wins, but by consistency, availability, and trust. Teams that remain healthy outperform teams that merely push harder. AI does not replace coaching wisdom—it sharpens it. It replaces guesswork with clarity and replaces reaction with foresight.

Ethics and responsibility remain inseparable from progress. As AI grows more powerful, the obligation to protect athlete autonomy, privacy, and dignity grows alongside it. The most successful systems are not those that control athletes, but those that empower them. Transparency, consent, and collaboration are not obstacles to innovation—they are the conditions that allow it to thrive.

Looking ahead, injury prevention will no longer exist as a separate discipline. It will be embedded into every decision—from training design to competition scheduling to career planning. Predictive ecosystems, digital twins, and real-time intelligence will guide athletes through entire careers with precision that once seemed impossible. Injury will not disappear, but surprise will.

The true legacy of AI injury prediction is not that athletes will never get hurt. It is that fewer careers will be defined by what could have been. Fewer seasons will end prematurely. Fewer athletes will be forced to choose between passion and health. The silent losses that once defined sport will become rarer, replaced by continuity and control.

As this book closes, the message is clear: peak performance is no longer about burning brightest—it is about lasting longest while still competing at the highest level. Intelligence, not recklessness, defines the new elite. Awareness replaces denial. Strategy replaces sacrifice.

The athletes who thrive in this era will not be those who ignore risk, but those who master it. They will train with confidence, compete with clarity, and retire knowing they extracted the full value of their potential without destroying the body that carried it.

This is the era of intelligent longevity. And it has already begun.

www.ingramcontent.com/pod-product-compliance
Lightning Source LLC
LaVergne TN
LVHW022023200926
848481LV00007B/2519